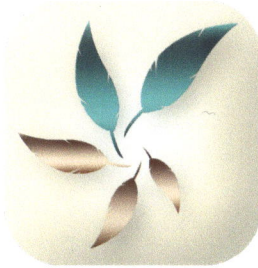

Manifested Blessings

Everyday People Share Their Manifesting
Stories and Secrets

Manifested Blessings

Everyday People Share Their Manifesting Stories and Secrets

JUDITH RICHARDSON SCHROEDER

Published by Carnelian Moon Publishing

www.carnelianmoonpublishing.com

Copyright © 2020 Judith Richardson Schroeder

Paperback ISBN: 978-1-989-707-04-3

eBook ISBN: 978-1-989-707-03-6

Printed in the United States of America

Contents

Prologue by *Judith Richardson Schroeder*   *1*

A Hole In My Heart by *Deborah Ann Davis*   *5*

Your Brilliance Is The Key by *Debbie Belnavis-Brimble*   *15*

Fur Baby Suzy by *Mary Ananda Shakti*   *25*

Manifesting Stories for Children by *Cathy Gagliardi*   *33*

The Light Within by *Winifred Adams*   *45*

As We Leave You by *Judith Richardson Schroeder*   *55*

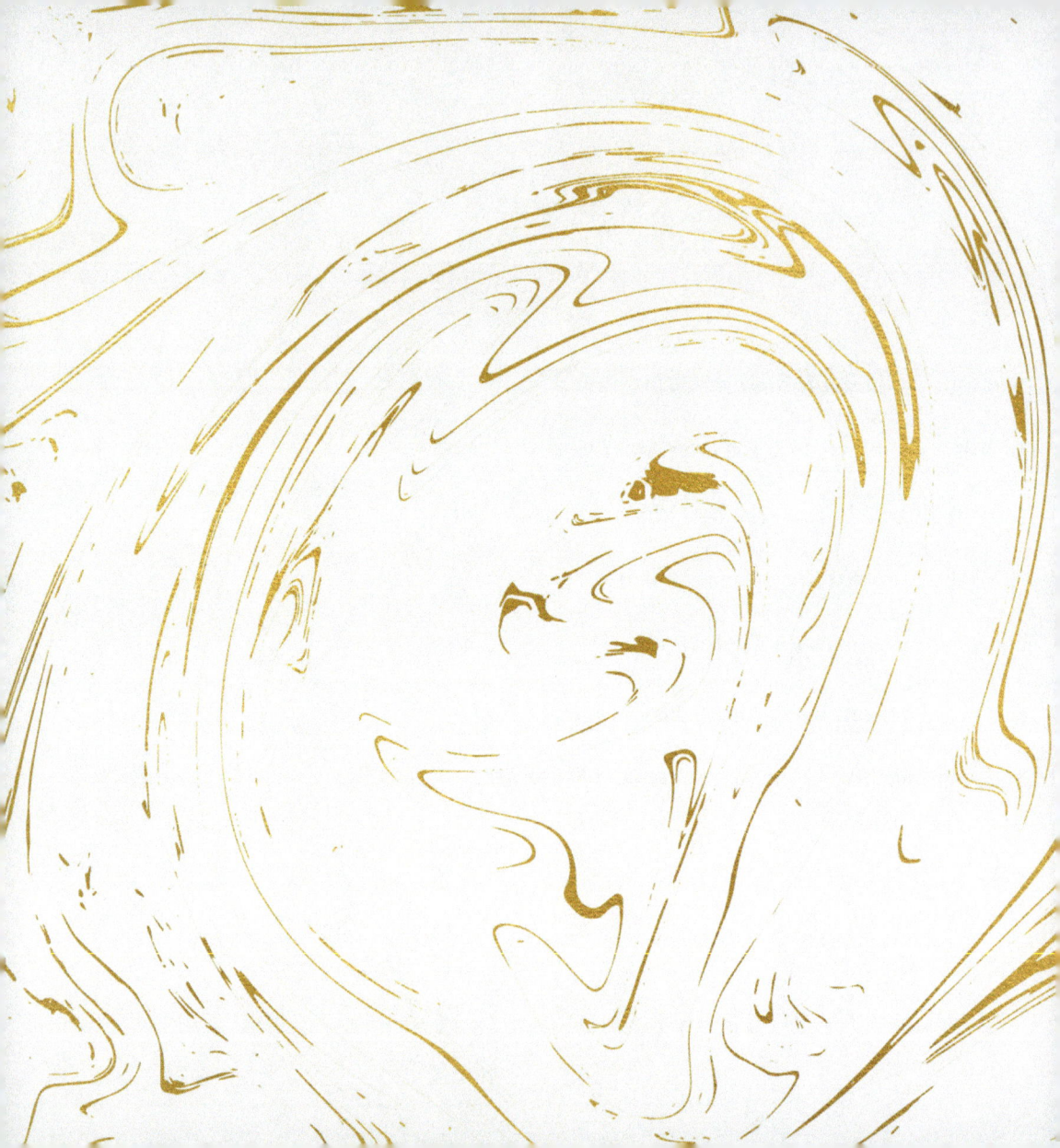

Prologue

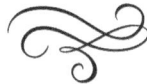

*I*T HAS ALWAYS been my intent to share stories of manifestations with, by, and for others. I am beyond honored to share with you the stories from the five incredible authors who have so generously shared their experiences with you in this beautiful volume of Manifested Blessings.

The act of creating is an inherent part of who we are as human beings, all of us being incredible creations ourselves. I hope the stories within the covers of this little book will touch your heart, ignite your Spirit, and encourage you to look to your own life to identify those beautiful moments of creative manifesting that you have been blessed to receive as well. We all have those moments. We are all powerful Creators in our own right. It is the hopes of myself and all the amazing authors of this beautiful little book, that you receive the gift of belief – and just like each of the wonderful stories shared here, that your belief in the power of YOU, shines through every single day as you walk through this world as the unique creator of your life's experiences.

If you have a story you'd like to share in an upcoming volume of Manifested Blessings, I hope you will reach out to me. I'd love to include your story in a future book. Reach me at publishme@carnelianmoonpublishing.com. If you enjoy these stories and would like to provide us with a review, please email your thoughts to us at reviews@carnelianmoonpublishing.com.

After enjoying these stories, we hope you will join us in our Online **TILA** community. The Inspired Living Academy (**TILA**) is where our authors have shared their additional content. It is a place where learning new ideas, practicing new skills and expanding your personal growth journey with us is accessed.

This immersive learning environment is always a work in progress and ever changing as content and authors are added with each of our new books. New Titles are in the works including more Manifested Blessings Volumes as well as a new series: Gifts of Gratitude. Future titles in The Inspired Living Anthologies includes *Spirit and Soul, Embracing Energy, Sacred Signs and Blessings,* and more to come!

The book you now have before you is meant to inspire you and move you forward, but it is also meant to support you in whatever your journey forward may look like to you. To visit us in our Online Community, The Inspired Living Academy, we have included a special QR-Code below. You will also be able to access via computer once you've become a member, and our community will remain accessible to you via your mobile phone for on the go visits with us! Once in our Online Community you will have access to additional content that the authors in this book are excited to share with you. Your membership in this Online community is FREE and provides you access to take part in upcoming workshops, webinars, events, and more! As future titles become available, additional communities will be made available to you with each book purchase.

 Simply use your smart phone to scan the QR-Code (or enter the site's address https://theinspiredlivingacademy.newzenler.com in the browser of your choice from your computer.). For QR-Code users, a password is required to gain access to the site from your mobile phone the first time you visit. QRPassword: tilabless.

Manifest Your Best Life by joining us soon. We can't wait to welcome you to the Community!

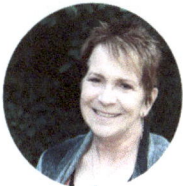 **Judith Richardson Schroeder**
Publisher
Carnelian Moon Publishing Inc.

4

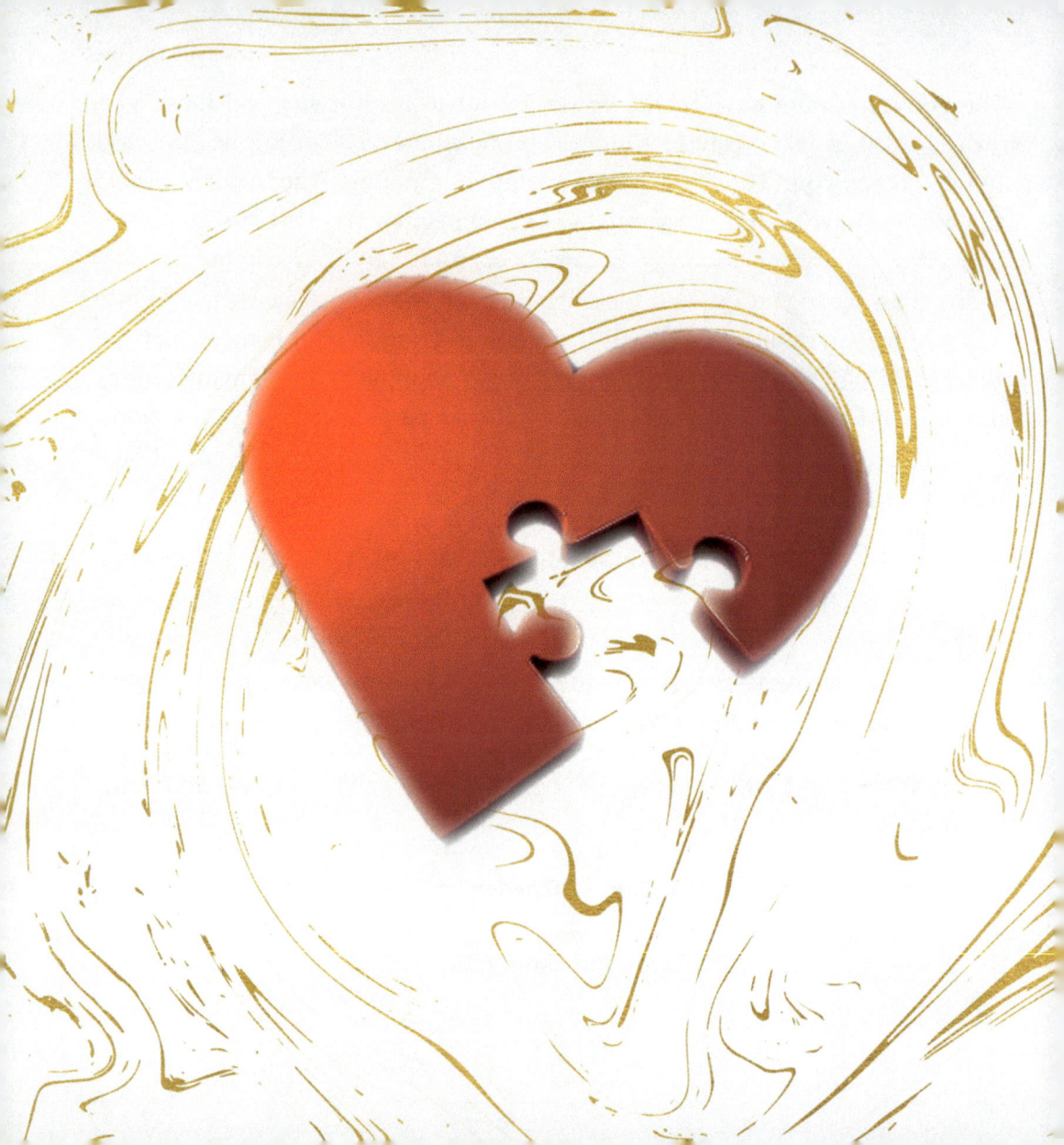

A Hole In My Heart

By Deborah Ann Davis

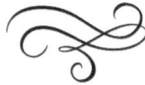

"What happens when people open their hearts?

They get better."

~Haruki Murakami

*S*TAIRS ABOVE ME… stairs below me.

Panting, I contemplated which way I should go from my seat on a middle step. No, this is not a metaphor for Life. This was me, an active, slender, 40-something mom, suddenly not able to make it all the way up one flight of stairs to my bedroom. I'd expected my Lyme disease to make me tired, but this seemed a little extreme.

Concern steered me toward the gym. It's a well-known fact that exercise and movement boost your immune system, so it made sense to add it to my anti-Lyme disease arsenal. Determined to slowly and gently help myself heal, I hired a personal trainer to guide me.

We began with the standard fitness assessments. The objective of the cardio test was to see how fast the heart recovered after exercise. It consisted of taking my starting pulse, stepping up and down for five minutes, then taking the pulse again, and then again, every minute until the heartbeat returned to normal. The objective is to see how fast the heart recovers after exercise.

I, of course, wasn't up to stepping for five minutes, so my trainer modified the test to just two minutes. After I dutifully stepped for two minutes, he checked my heart rate a second time. "Um, your pulse is lower than before the test."

I stopped swigging my water. "That doesn't make any sense. I'm still catching my breath." His frown worried me. "Maybe you made a mistake. Let's try it again."

After a brief rest, we tested again… and once again my heart rate dropped following exercise.

"What does that mean?" I quavered.

"It means we can't work together until you see a cardiologist and get medically cleared."

Let the Tests Begin!

Having my very own heart doctor seemed like an overkill solution for getting up the stairs, but I found one with some serious credentials who agreed to take me on.

Blood work. Echocardiograms. Ultrasounds. Stress tests. EKGs. Monitors I carried around with me. With all those tests, the cardiologist still spent a lot of time listening to my heart with a stethoscope.

Eventually, he informed me that I had a hole in my heart.

Specifically, it was in my septum (the wall that separates the left and right sides of the heart). The hole accounted for the odd noises the doctor kept hearing. Fortunately, he told me, this type of hole could be repaired surgically by putting a patch over it and letting heart cells grow over that.

Fortunately?

That wasn't all. The tests showed my pulse dropping to 37 beats a minute. No wonder I was so tired.

The doctor's solution? I needed a pacemaker.

A pacemaker? My weak little heart thumped in alarm. "I thought those were for old people!"

"It's unusual because you're young. However, we'll have to wait until they cure your Lyme disease."

"Wait a minute. I need to exercise to help fight my Lyme disease, but I need the Lyme disease gone before I can get a pacemaker to allow me to exercise?" I was trying to be calm, but, "That's crazy! How am I supposed to get better?"

"Get plenty of rest."

Seriously?

While You Wait

Does anyone know a sick mom who has time to rest?

Mornings I acted peppy until my daughter left for school. I slept until the early afternoon, waking in time to grocery shop before she returned. I'd fake an abundance of energy until she disappeared to do her homework and then I'd sink onto the couch until she emerged a couple of hours later. After a quick snack, we'd hit the hay (me gratefully, and her with youthful resentment).

One day, I chatted with a woman while she easily rearranged wooden boxes at a farm stand. Apparently, we had both had Lyme disease. Seeing her so strong nudged me to ask, "How long did it take you to get over it?"

"I'm not over it. This is just a good day. I spend bad days on the couch. I've had it for two years."

Two years? My insides froze. All these weeks I'd just assumed I'd get better once the disease ran its course. I was not going to spend the next two years of my life hoping for a "good day." *No way!*

Taking Things into My Own Hands

I didn't care what the doctor said. What sense did it make to just rest and wait to get better? Every fiber of my being told me to keep moving for my body's sake. I fell back on my teacher credo: It's better to ask forgiveness than permission. Soooo… I defiantly dragged myself around the gym, dodging the personal trainer.

I slowly walked on the treadmill for about 20-second increments and then rested until I felt ready to try it again.

I used very small free weights (Did you know they make one-pound dumbbells?) because the machine weights were too much for me.

I practiced going up the bedroom stairs, visualizing doing the entire flight without stopping.

I figured my body needed all the support I could give it. I drank lots of water and did my best to eat healthy foods.

I also visualized those little spirochetes being annihilated by my immune system in my hostile, antibiotic-infested body.

A Surgical Alternative

Determined to explore everything, I turned to my father. He had once told me how he avoided hemorrhoids surgery by instructing his body to heal itself. My dad had theorized if we were in charge of our brains/minds, and our minds were in charge of our bodies, he only had to give his mind a focused order to *heal* his body.

At the time, I was skeptical, but now…well, what could it hurt?

Why wait for heart cells to grow over some surgical patch? Why not get them started now? If my dad could encourage his body to heal, so could I.

Every night, I folded my hands across my chest and sent healing energy to my septum. Strangely, my hands would heat up, giving me a focal point as I imagined this as healing energy.

Sometimes I told the cells around the hole to multiply until it sealed up. I also told my circulatory system to carry the necessary components my cells needed. Frequently I sent generic healing energy to the entire heart, plus all the blood vessels leading to and from it. And, I asked my other organs to help in every way possible. I mean, why not?

I didn't know what I was doing. I just made it up as I went along. I figured every little bit would help, and it certainly couldn't hurt to concentrate on healing.

Besides, a Red Cross First Aid instructor had shared a story about a woman who saved her husband's life when he suffered a heart attack. She didn't know CPR, except for what she'd seen in movies. She alternated pushing on his chest, blowing into his mouth, and screaming for help from their living room, until a neighbor heard her and called 911. She didn't know what she was doing, either, but she kept him alive by doing anything she could think of, and he lived to tell the story.

That was my intention—to try anything I could think of to focus on my heart. And guess what?

It Worked!

By the time I recovered from Lyme disease a couple of months later, my heart rate was on the lower side, but definitely within the normal range, rendering the pacemaker solution obsolete. *Yay!* The cardiologist never figured out what had happened to my heart, but eventually, he stopped watching for a health reversal. My monthly visits became quarterly, then every six months, and finally, yearly.

Presently, I see him every three years. Usually I have an echocardiogram (the test that originally revealed the hole in my heart). The hole stopped showing up on their tests years ago. That's right. It's gone, my septum's sealed, and no one had to crack open my chest. I wanted my body to heal, and incredibly, it did.

I believe being on antibiotics for four months is what messed with my heart. I've had Lyme disease twice since that scary period ten years ago, but under the care of a naturopath, herbal extracts and supplements have cured me, not antibiotics; and I have had no heart problems since.

A coincidence? I think not. ;-)

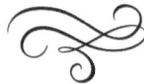

Deborah Ann Davis, Award-winning Author, Educator and Trainer, Founder of The Awesome Mom Tribe.

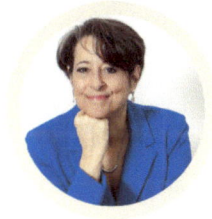

Deborah Ann has helped countless families navigate the tumultuous teen years. As producer of a successful teenage daughter, and a former teenager herself, this middle/high school teacher distills three decades of experience into exciting live events and insightful books. Her timely information on effective communication, emotional health, and physical wellbeing helps moms foster positive, healthy relationships within their families.

Connect with Deborah:

http://deborahanndavis.com

http://awesomemomtribe.com

https://www.facebook.com/AwesomeMomTribe

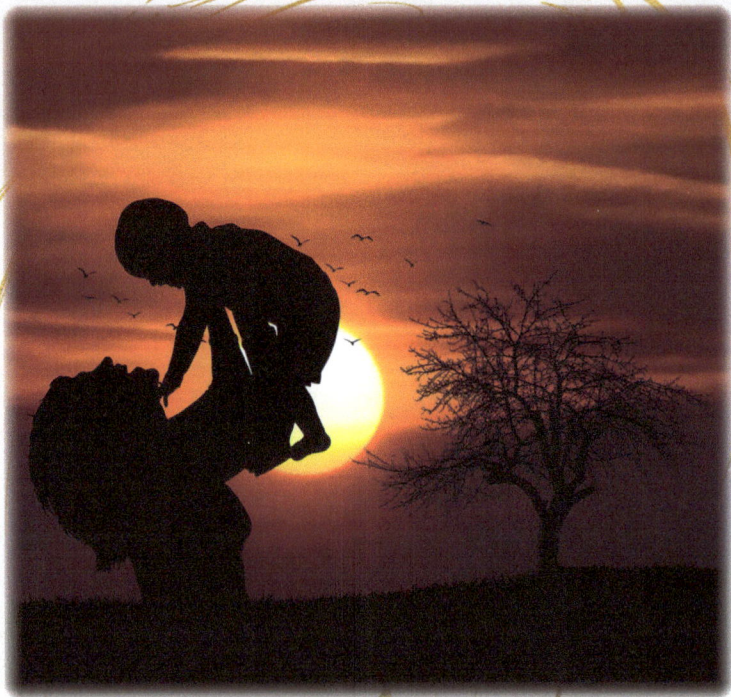

Your Inner Brilliance is Key to Your Manifestation Superpower

By Debbie Belnavis-Brimble

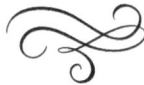

"Your job is to let your light shine brightly!"

~ Lisa Nichols

*B*E CAREFUL WHAT you ask for; you might end up getting exactly that, and then some ….. although it's not always in the form that you expected.

My life has been filled with blessings, as I like to call them. Little did I know as I got older, I would realize these blessings were manifestations. I had called them into my own life with the support of God, Universe, and Source (GUS). You see, in my 20s and early 30s, I had no idea about this airy-fairy stuff – how naive was I back then? The word manifestation didn't feature in my vocabulary. It wasn't until I had my son, and I took time to reflect through my life and embraced my new way of thinking and believing.

As I reflected on those moments during my life, growing up as a child initially in England and then in Jamaica, there were many occasions I can draw upon where I manifested exactly what I wanted without even realizing it.

I was a timid and overly reserved child, preferring to be in the background, yet that was never God's plan for me. He had a divine plan that I had no idea would materialize in the way it has.

Unexpected and amazing things happened. I became the President of Key Club at the age of 15; at the time, I was the youngest president at my school up to that point. I was so proud of myself. When I started my first job at 17, rather than going to the sixth form, I wondered if it was a mistake. However, I was never a scholar, so I welcomed the opportunity to start earning an income. About six months on the job, I was the youngest member of the team in a newly opened shipping company. I was working with colleagues two and three times my age, yet there were conversations taking place about me becoming the supervisor. The only challenge: I was so much younger. Although this didn't happen, I was honored they saw something in me that I didn't see in myself at the time.

The trend followed me because years later, when I started working at a law firm in the UK as a legal secretary at the age of 20, I quickly became the senior member of the team. This trend continued to show up throughout my life as I earned promotion after promotion after promotion.

I was a born leader and didn't even notice or appreciate it until years later. Looking back now, I realize my real superpower has always been creating LOVE CONNECTIONS with others effortlessly. I didn't always fully appreciate or value it.

I fostered meaningful connections with others through love. The flashbacks, along my timeline of life, showed me all the meaningful connections along my journey. With each reminder, my heart warmed more and more. That's when it clicked; positive blessings entered my life when I had meaningful connections and shared the love with others!

There was one special love connection when I was about 15. I attended an orphanage in Kingston, Jamaica. We had a drive to collect donations of clothing, non-perishable food items, toiletries, and other items. We spent some time with the children and played with them, read to them, and it was a beautiful experience. There was a one-year-old baby boy there that I had an instant connection with. He was the most amazing little soul, and I remember thinking that these children deserved so much more than they had and the standard of living they had. My heart cried just witnessing the environment and the lack of tenderness and love, especially for the babies. I wanted to pick all the crying babies up and share my love with them.

I recall rushing home and asking my parents if we could adopt this baby boy I met. I fell in love with him. I fell in love with all children that day, and my passion for becoming a mother began.

I had a passion and love for children my entire life. So much so, I remember one of my Mom's friends saying I loved children so much that someone like me may never end up having children! She based that on her witnessing other women who had astounding mother instincts but were unable to have children for various reasons, including health reasons. That stayed with me for most of my life. As the years passed by, I began to accept this as my truth. Being in a relationship with someone for over seven years, I was desperate to expand and share the love I had inside of me with a child. It wasn't time, though.

I am so grateful that God, Universe, and Source (GUS) understood the time was not right. The gift I manifested years later through true love and soul connection is what my heart truly desired. Even when I was prepared to settle back then, my superpower was at work protecting my heart and soul.

Within seven months of ending that relationship, I came to realize my soul connection had been right in front of me for the past ten years. But I hadn't recognized it. I had been content in my relationship and fully committed, not interested in another direction. When that relationship ended, it became clear. GUS had placed me with someone who was never suitable for me to support me in truly tapping into what I knew I wanted in my soul love connection.

My husband was always there, always in my life, and the love connection had already begun ten years prior. The relationship was already divinely orchestrated, all I had to do was enjoy the process. Five years later, we were married, and of course, the nurturing motherly instincts were even more present. I was in a soul connected relationship, so of course, this is the moment where my little boy was meant to find his parents. At the age of 38, when I started to disconnect myself from the outcome of becoming a mother, we finally got the news that we were expecting our gift from God.

These are just two powerful manifestations around calling in my family. There have been so many more, including many promotions, starting my very first business, numerous qualifications, amazing business opportunities, relocating from England to the USA, and more!

With all of these fruitful blessings, there have been several steps that have always been present — combined with my superpower of LOVE CONNECTIONS.

Now, I want to share my **Inner Brilliance Blessing Process** with you.

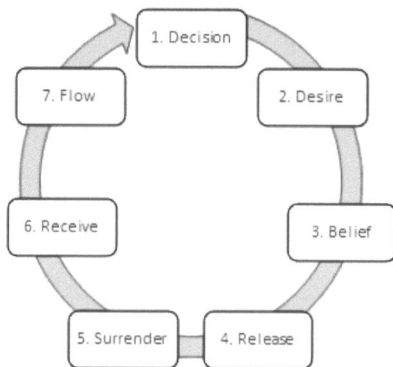

These steps have supported my journey and they can support yours too.

1.   Decision

from a place of knowing comes your desire to implement positive change in your life. Here you decide to implement this change even if you have no idea what it is or even where to start. All you need do is decide.

2.   Desire

is vital. A burning desire is gained by tapping into what you truly want to bring into your life to elevate your successes and bring you clarity. Spend the time to explore and define your desires fully.

3. Release

everything that works against your ultimate desire, including your limiting beliefs which no longer serve you. Carry out a process of release by writing down everything you are letting go of. Then create your new story, write a new reality you are aiming to achieve.

4. Believe

in an undeniable faith in GUS and yourself, knowing and embracing that you have the most amazing inner brilliance and you deserve to receive what your heart truly desires. Believe with your entire body, using all your senses – see it, hear it, feel it, smell it, and even taste it if it applies. Embody your inner knowing from deep within that you already have whatever your heart truly desires.

5. Surrender

Most people think of surrendering as giving up, submitting, or being defeated. I tend to lean to a more positive take.

You already know you have an undeniable belief that your desires are already within your reality. Now, surrender to GUS with complete trust and allow the inevitable to take place. Release worry, fear, guilt, or any other emotion that prevents you from entirely calling in your desires.

6. Receive

From a place of knowing that you have already received your heart's desires and be open to that receiving. Be open to the possibilities that you are already receiving what you desire. Be ready to receive from a place of love, honoring yourself fully.

7. Flow

You have fully embraced the decision, desire, release, belief, surrendering, and receiving. Now, from a place of **FLOW**, you have arrived where all you desire is already yours. You have proven that your superpowers support your success. It's time to just **BE**.

With your superpowers and combined manifesting elements bringing your desires into reality, it's time to dig deep. Embrace all the magic from the blessings that already exist in your life! And, all those that are just around the corner being revealed to you right now. Be open to the possibilities and remember, you have incredible superpowers. Permit yourself to use them!

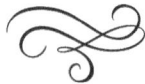

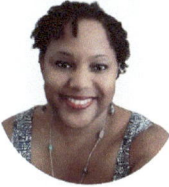

Debbie Belnavis-Brimble, Founder of The Inner Brilliance Academy & Co-Founding Publisher of Carnelian Moon Publishing.

Debbie supports women worldwide tapping into their inner brilliance, embracing their true selves and sharing their truth. Women partnering with Debbie achieve success in:

- Reconnect with their own inner brilliance
- Learn to love themselves like never before
- Regain confidence
- Live the life you truly desire with purpose, passion and possibility.

Connect with Debbie:

www.innerbrillianceacademy.com

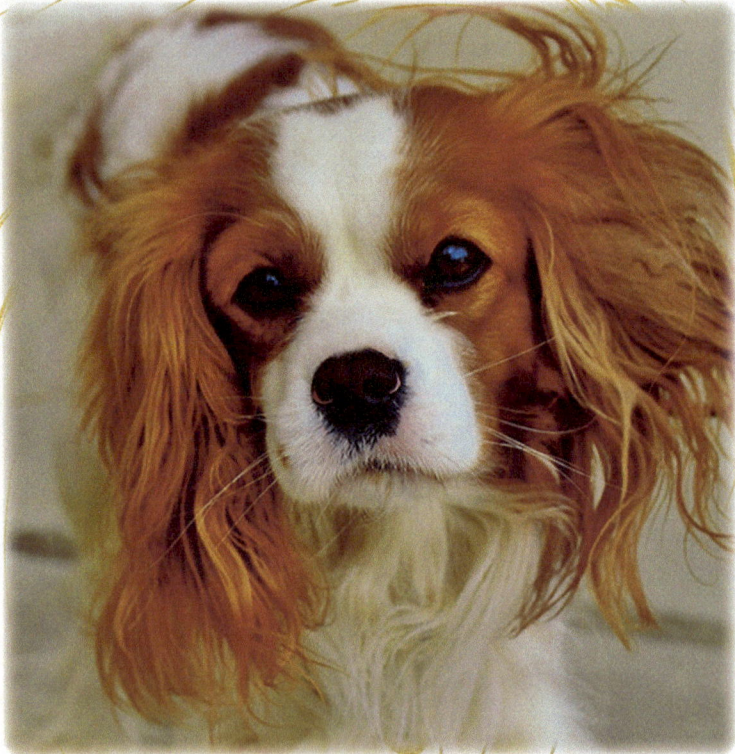

My Fur Baby Suzy

By Mary Ananda Shakti

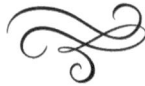

"Dogs are not our whole life, but they make our lives whole."

~Roger Caras

*I*T WAS FEBRUARY 1994, just a normal day. My three kids were gone to school. I was pottering about the house doing the daily chores when a thought which surprised me came into my mind. It surprised me because before this we never thought of nor discussed getting a dog, but that's what my mind said, "get a dog", and not just any dog but a Cavalier King Charles. I didn't know anyone who had one, so it wasn't as if I was even familiar with them or crossed paths with one. But I did know what they looked like so I could imagine the big eyes and long ears.

I got the Buy and Sell magazine and looked up the pet section. I found a two-year-old for sale which was in Kerry. As I lived in County Mayo at the time, I told the lady I would be in Limerick, which was closer, for Easter and that I would give her a call and if she still had him, I would come for him.

The Big Bang

Well, Easter came, and yes, I was in Limerick. After a walkabout town where I picked up the auto trade magazine because I was thinking of changing my car, I set off for my sister's house to bring Easter eggs for her children when it happened. My twelve-year-old son was with me in the car as we sat and waited for the traffic lights to turn green at a very busy crossroads. We chatted away as the music was playing and then the lights changed. As I pulled out, I saw out of the corner of my eye a car speeding towards us. I told my son to hold tight. We were going to be hit. And then the big bang crash! Everything was now in slow motion; we were like rag dolls inside the car as it bounced around. My head was banging off my window!

My Guardian Angel

I was now facing north instead of East. People were coming from all directions to see if we were ok. One man seemed like he was taking care of me. He stood with his hands on the top of the door. I felt like I couldn't move, and even if I wanted to, he wasn't going to let me. He said, "the driver is coming back now," then he asked if my neck was ok. It felt like his calming voice was bringing me back into my body as my head had been banged and shook about a lot.

When the driver did come to the car, he asked if we could settle up now as the guards (police) were coming. I was able to ask what we were settling for when he said, "the damage to my car!" I then said, "what about my son and me? We don't know what damage is done to us!" I found out later that the man who was taking care of me like my guardian angel was an accident investigator. I was blessed to have him there taking charge as I may have got out to find my son if he hadn't stood so close to the door until the ambulance came. He was protecting me.

During it all, I realized my son was missing from the car, yet there was no broken windscreen, and the door was closed. I began to panic as he didn't know anyone in the area. Where could he be? I asked the people standing beside the car if they had seen him and no one had. And then he just got back into the car, and he told me he had followed the other driver up the road to get the license number just in case he didn't stop. Then I realized the music was playing in the car. It was a tape that just went on and on.

The ambulance came and took both of us to the hospital. Once again, I fretted as I couldn't see my son in the ambulance nor at the hospital, but I was assured he was there, and that he was fine. We were released later in the evening only to find out my car was a write-off and not worth fixing. So, with all that going on, I had forgotten about the Cavalier King Charles in Kerry. In fact, I totally forgot that I had even wanted a dog.

As the weeks went on, I found myself slipping into a deep state of depression with suicidal thoughts. Only for having my children depending on me I may have carried it through. Now I had no choice but to seek my doctor's help. I was a single mom with three teenagers, and I wasn't coping well at all. I was sad and crying all the time. It wasn't easy on them, and it caused a lot of confusion. I was referred to a psychiatrist who told me I had reactive depression which had been brought on by the accident. He then prescribed Prozac. He also sent me for daily counseling to talk about the car accident until I was sick of listening to myself. Just about then the Prozac began to work, and I had my first positive thought in months. Life finally began to improve again.

Along Came the Cavalier

One day in the middle of summer, I was collecting my daughter from her friend's house. While I was waiting, a dog I had never seen or heard about before came over and was crawling up my legs begging for me to say hello. It was a Cavalier King Charles. Just then, my daughter told me they were giving away the dog, and she asked if I wanted to take her home. An instant connection was made between us. Of course, I wanted to give her a home! I was invited into the house, and once again, the dog that I was now told was called Suzy was climbing up my leg again. I learned from her owners that it wasn't normal behavior for her as she usually nipped at visitor's heels. They asked if I wanted her and you can guess my answer.

I brought her home, and the following day I dropped her off at the grooming lady. When I went back to collect her, she got so excited to see me that when I said I only had her for one day, the lady was amazed. I know we made a connection back in February when I had first had that thought about getting a dog, come into my mind. Somehow the connection was made through my daughter who regularly visited her friend and owned Suzy, the Cavalier King Charles dog all along.

Suzy and I became such good and close friends sharing so much together. We strolled the roads and beaches together. She was a faithful family pet whom we all loved. My family is all grown with children of their own now, but they often talk about the things we did together with Suzy. I also witnessed her nipping at my friend's heels when they came to visit. She was a cheeky lady, indeed.

The Transformation

I was still working through depression on Prozac when we first owned Suzy. Morning time was hardest as the day ahead seemed very long to get through. Suzy sat on my lap through it all. If I sat all day, she would sit with me. We were inseparable and went everywhere together. Then the day came when I realized Prozac had taken me as far as it could, and I needed to reach out and find my way of healing myself. That's when I discovered that some individuals I knew from a business aspect were healers. I went to them weekly and began to feel much stronger. I weaned myself off Prozac and was now living happily again with Suzy and my children. I felt then if I could come through all that with support, then I could support others to do the same. That's when I chose to become a Holistic Therapist and teacher.

In January of 1996, I was booked to go with a group on a spiritual journey to India. Just before I left Suzy got ill, I called the vet who medicated her. He didn't say it was serious. He thought it was just a bug. But this was her time to go as she crossed the rainbow bridge while I was away and perhaps, she knew just how difficult I would find our goodbye. It's as if she knew her work was done. We had loved each other unconditionally for only a short time, but Suzy is unforgettable and loved forever. And, I firmly believe she was the blessing I was meant to manifest at that difficult time in my life, and I'm grateful for the time she spent with us.

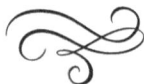

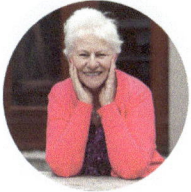

Mary Ananda Shakti, Life and Laughter Coach, Bliss Energy Therapist.

Mary supports people worldwide in realizing their authentic selves as their inner happiness emerges whilst allowing their fountain of bliss to flow. Through teamwork your confidence shall soar and your limitations will dissolve. You shall feel more love, compassion and gratitude for yourself and others.

Mary inspires people and shares the teaching tools with them, allowing them to live the life of their dreams.

Connect with Mary:

https://laughteryogaireland.org
https://hypnosisdonegal.com

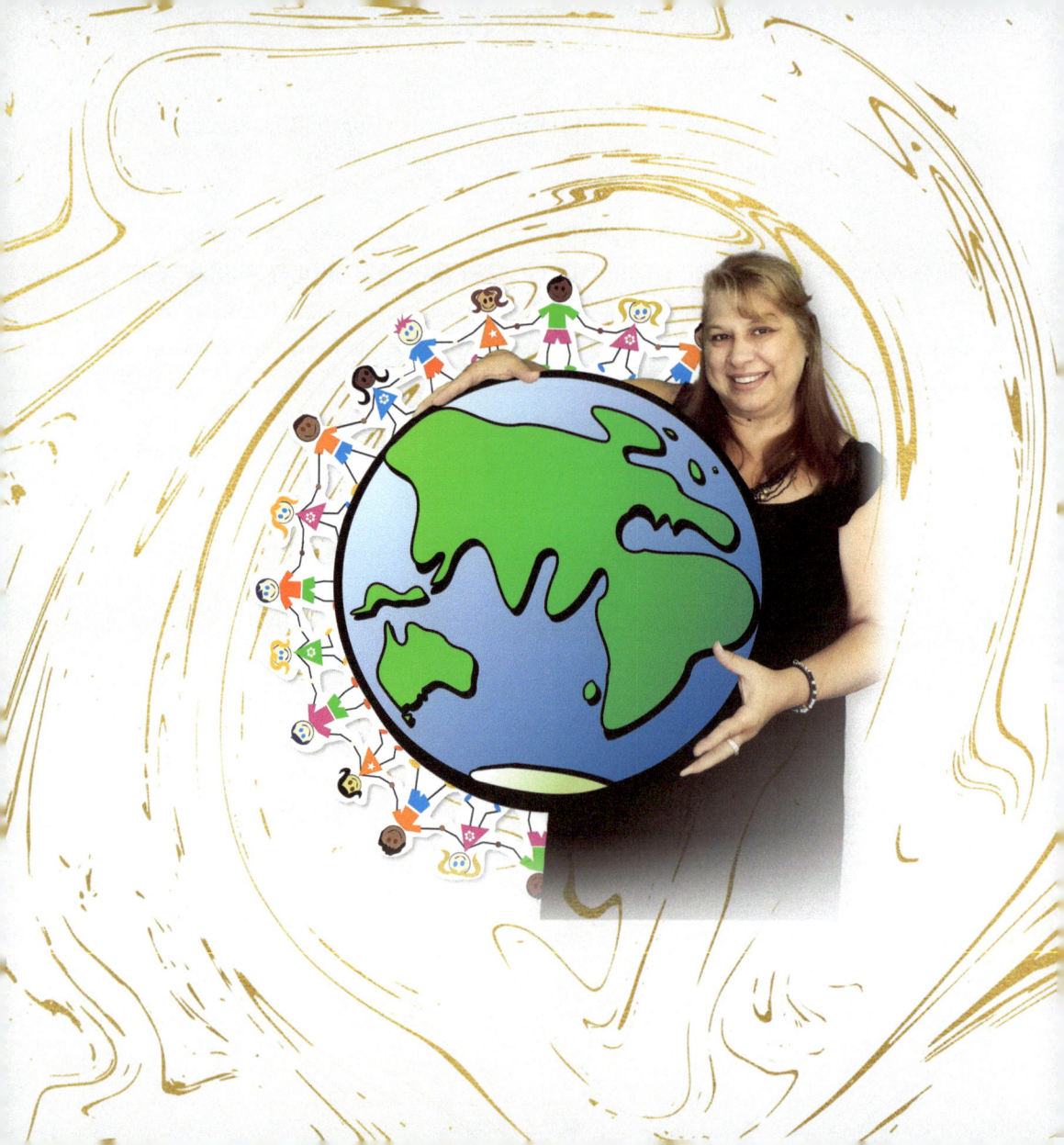

Manifesting Stories For Children

By Cathy Gagliardi

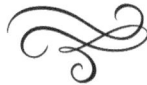

"A person is only limited by the thoughts that he chooses."

~ James Allen

ANIFESTING ... WHAT is manifesting anyway? Manifesting is to ask for something for yourself.

Asking for something for myself is greedy, selfish and unacceptable.

Hmmm, let's rethink this whole process!

Manifesting: To involve the Universe in the pursuit of your goals and always trust that it will be for your highest good.

Since we have been instructed by society to give of ourselves, not expect anything from others, and never ask for anything if we want to be good people, it is very difficult to understand this process and realize how important it is.

One step at a time. It is almost like unlearning everything I thought would bring me satisfaction and joy. Then I realized that to have real joy in my life I needed to take a look at myself from an outside point of view. It was not who I wanted to be at all. It occurred to me that I had no idea how to be that person.

The question went through my head continuously, "Who am I and who do I want to be?"

The answer slowly became clear to me. I wanted to help people and spread love. Ok, that was the easy part but at the time it was a real effort to just get myself to that point.

Who Am I Meant to Be?

I remember as clearly as if it was yesterday. I stood outside my house after work. Before heading in, I looked up to the amazing Hamilton sunset and made a wish. I wanted to be a vessel for loving, healing energy from the Universe. To tell you the truth, I was not even sure what I was asking for. I wanted to heal all the sick people in the world. I wanted to make everyone feel loved: all my family, friends, acquaintances, those who lived on my street, everyone I passed as I drove to the mall, everyone in the mall, all their families and friends. The list went on until I got overwhelmed and started to cry. I knew it was impossible...or...was...it?

I began frequently making this wish and frequently sent love to all those around me.

One grey, miserable day as I started work, I began to feel awful. I noticed everyone felt the same way, crabby and complaining or rude, and there was an overall darkness hanging over us. When I went home for lunch, I thought about how heavy I felt and how little I had accomplished. What if I did an experiment?

When I went back to work in the afternoon, everyone was the same but now they also carried the after-lunch heaviness. Without outwardly showing it, I decided and intended to spread love. Everyone I encountered got a huge blast of love energy. Haha, I laughed to myself knowing how silly I was being. Nevertheless, I went around to all the offices and every cubicle and spread love to every corner of the building. Slowly the darkness lifted, and I could hear laughter, see smiles and watch people helping one another. This transformation passed from the receptionist to the folks entering the building. I really didn't trust that the attitude change was due to loving thoughts coming from my heart. I did know though, that I just wanted to revel in the idea of it all.

Guess what? I was addicted to this reaction and I made certain I practiced spreading love to everyone in this way as often as possible.

During another average day, while working in my cubicle, my hands started to tingle and heat up when my desk partner began talking about the pain she was carrying in her back. For some reason I had a strong urge to put my hands on her, but I knew that might come across as just weird. I did start following my feelings, though and without having any idea what was going on, I helped ease people's painful backs, necks and other physical discomforts wherever I laid my hands. I was nervous I may be doing something wrong, yet I felt obligated to try to heal everyone.

It was suggested that I take Reiki courses which I did, studying Reiki 1 and Reiki 11. Learning that it wasn't me who was doing the healing, but our combined energy or Universal energy took the pressure off me and let me just do what I felt led to do. I haven't felt the desire to do this for money, but I still shyly ask people in pain if they mind if I put my hands on them.

I am learning more and more about this mysterious world which I really can't describe in words. Trusting is hard for me, but when I let my resistance down and become receptive to the beautiful energies that swirl around, it always manages to surprise and awe me.

Discovering My Gifts

During a very dark time in my life, I found a need for guidance. I had tried to manifest a better life but didn't know what was meant by that. Being unclear, even in my own head had me going in circles. I finally asked not just for guidance but a clear answer for what I should do.   No clues or vague indications would do. Just then, before my very eyes and in front of my car was a butterfly. That's cute, I thought. This butterfly flew in front of me on the driver's side of my car all the way to my mother's home. Suddenly, I knew I needed to be there. That was the clear answer. It was the place I would feel all the comfort and calmness that would eventually open the doors to reveal the person I have been working to become.

As I begin to acknowledge the need for following the path that will most benefit myself and the world, I can visualize the steppingstones that are leading the way.

I am learning that bringing energy to a higher vibration in my life results in real life miracles.

After I had my second child, I was desperately trying to discover what it was that I wanted to do with my life. When asked what it was that would make me feel fulfilled, the only answer that came out of my mouth was, "I want to touch children." People laughed and I did too. I didn't really have any words for this feeling and didn't have a clue as to what that meant. I researched physiotherapy classes but at that time they were only available in Toronto and Buffalo. Both unacceptable locations for a young mother with two young children. Next, I thought I could work or somehow be a part of the local children's hospital even if it was as a volunteer. That was an easy solution.

I ventured out on a beautiful sunny day, confident and excited with my idea. I was not sure what I had to offer but I was willing to do anything, and a phone call just wouldn't do. So off I went. I practically bounced through the doors of the hospital and announced that I wanted to be a part of these children's lives. I wanted to apply for a job or volunteer. When I was asked what my skill set was, I stumbled and could only say, "I love children". Haha, now that I recall this conversation, it was pretty funny. When asked what it was I wanted to do, I blurted out the words, "I want to touch children!!!"

Oh brother, did I actually say that? Again?

After chatting a bit, the supervisor told me she recognized my enthusiasm and she thought I had a special gift to share. There was a group of children heading down for some reading time, and she asked if I would like to join them. These children were supervised and each of them lived with spina bifida and other very serious issues. They were also so excited to have a new face even though a stranger among them. No matter what they were going through they were just beautiful, unpredictable, silly and clever cherubs. They ranged in age, and all couldn't wait to snuggle up for a story. I hugged them one by one and sat with one child on my lap. My heart exploded. We laughed and played, and they completely wore me out. I couldn't erase the smile from my face.

After my time was finished, I walked past the front desk and said goodbye to the ladies there. They shared a very important message with me that I knew I was meant to hear. "Do whatever you have to do to be a part of children's lives. It is necessary that your gift be shared."

Wow, I thought that was so nice of them to say that. I was walking on air. I could barely fit my huge head into the car.

From Tragedy Comes Healing

I sat in my car and reflected on that little piece of heaven I had just experienced. Then it happened. Tears came pouring down my face as I sobbed like a baby. Totally helpless to stop the overwhelming feeling of guilt that suddenly swept over me! I had two healthy children. How would I be able to leave these children and go home to mine without feeling I had been changed by them and this experience? It's not that I didn't appreciate my kiddos every single day, I did. Maybe it was not guilt. Maybe it was sadness. I'm still not too sure. I wanted to help these children however I could, but what about all the other children of the world that need help, health care, food, clean water, education, a safe place to live, someone to take care and be responsible for them and love them? Too much to think about. More tears. If only I could find a way to touch children of the world more easily. I was manifesting again.

Today, I touch little lives through the stories I write for children and I put my whole heart and soul into making my books available to children and parents worldwide.

My first book, Bellyflies, was born from a sad tragedy. My dear friend who I just love to be in the presence of was hurting so badly. She had lost her oldest son to suicide. Without truly knowing how he felt, my heart broke for the pain her son and now her family was experiencing. Shock, emptiness and confusion are only some of the feelings that left me numb. I can't even begin to fathom what my friend and her family were experiencing. The emotions and reactions while still trying to function as a family are beyond me. I could only offer my friendship.

The night after I learned of the tragedy, I spent the evening unable to sleep. Instead, I wrote Bellyflies, a book that today helps children describe their feelings of anxiety, sadness, anger and upset more easily to the adults in their lives.

My vision is to create stories that help children learn tricks to identify, accept and deal with unfavourable emotions as they grow. My stories help children and parents connect in conversations and do so naturally and from the heart. My Manifested Blessings continue to not only bless me but especially the children of the world.

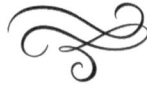

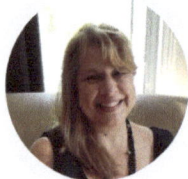

Cathy Gagliardi, Beloved Children's Author, Illustrator and International Speaker.

Cathy currently enjoys being surrounded at her home with her mom close by, enjoying the beauty of nature near Hamilton, Ontario, Canada. Her sons, Patrick and Gregory, encourage her big dreams!

Cathy is the author of several books helping children deal with anxiety and develop compassion for others while learning to accept themselves.

Connect with Cathy:

https://twinklinglynx.com

https://www.facebook.com/TwinklingLynx-2479264172118444/

twinklinglynx@gmail.com

This page is intentionally left blank

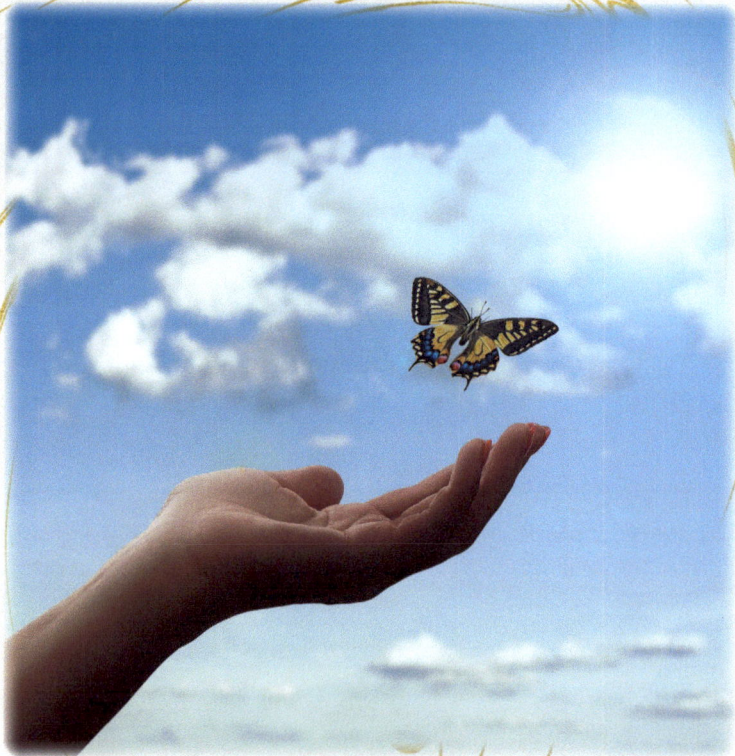

The Light Within Revealed in Silence

By Winifred Adams

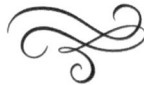

"Within each of us, there is silence. A silence as vast as the universe. And when we experience that silence, we remember who we are."

~ Gunilla Norris

*I*NTO THE SILENCE - When I began my spiritual journey, I was furious with the world. I had just graduated from high school, and a recent set of events upended my entire world, making me question everything in it.

As a child, I inherently understood and sensed things that most people don't see or feel. Whenever I'd share my 'creativity' with friends or my family, they thought I was strange. Yet, deep within me, I knew there was something more to life, and I knew without a shadow of a doubt that my life had a meaningful purpose. Most of all, however, I knew in my heart that all life had a meaningful purpose, even if I didn't see the adults aligning their actions to their words.

When my world turned upside down after high school graduation, I was at a boiling point. It was then that I made a bold decision and placed my college career on hold, deferred my education for a year, and went into silence for six months.

During my time of silence, I set out to find the answers to the questions that lingered in my heart. If I could see a world that seemingly no one else around me could see or feel, one of two things were true; either I was crazy, or they didn't know what I saw. I set out to prove the latter.

Before tofu was commonly in grocery stores and kale juice was a way of life, I was requesting Wegman's grocery store carry vegetarian products. My parents were embarrassed by me, and honestly didn't know what to do with me. I seemed like an alien to their world and their societal conditioning. Sometimes I'd feel great compassion for what I considered to be their lack of understanding, and other times I'd become very frustrated by their unwillingness to see beyond their limitations.

That year, I settled into my silence willingly, out of defiance to the world around me as well as to quiet all the voices coming at me telling me who to be, how to act, and what to think. I had to sort out my own feelings and hear my own inner voice which was drowning in a sea of opinions around me.

The Wisdom of Others

Before the internet was everyone's go-to, I would go to the bookstore and find anything I could on psychics, paranormal, and past life activity. I was led, one book after another to dig further into finding the truth behind what I could automatically see or feel. Where I grew up, there simply wasn't anyone I could talk to about these things, and I was tired of being called 'weird.'

Each book I read would give me more to consider about life after death, spirituality, and where our soul goes and who we are. But most importantly, I began to realize more about why we are here on Earth.

In typical Sagittarian fashion, I was eager to seek out the truth. I wanted the answers, and I wanted them from the Source! I wouldn't take no for an answer and proceeded to read the entire metaphysical section of the library in my hometown, which also included eastern philosophy and medical books relating to case histories that included medical intuition before it was given a name.

When I exhausted that avenue, I turned to the bookstores once again, following threads to special order books by Ruth Montgomery, Dick Sutphen, and any others I could get my hands on, including the channelings by SETH. In my hometown, the only 'channel' we knew of was a TV channel. All this was new to me, and yet somehow it resonated deeply with my heart as a kind of truth.

Soon I was learning about past-life regressions and the beauty of the spirit world, including the unconditional love that is always coming to us from beyond. As I researched and studied, I felt an ever-growing connection that was both comforting and necessary. At that point, I felt very alone in this world and found my guides and spirit friends/relatives a new, close ally in my daily activity.

The Arrival of Sam

As I settled into fall that year, I longed for a companion. Trying on my new skills of asking spirit for help, I ordered up a cat to be delivered. One afternoon I sat, silently, at lunch with my father, the energy thick in the air, when we both jumped as a loud 'THUD' hit the side porch door. There, with nails holding on and dug into the window frame was a cat peering in at us! This cat's appearance was perhaps one of the most unlikely events that might ever suddenly happen to anyone. We both craned to see, and sure enough, it really was a cat hanging there looking in at us.

Silently, I jumped for joy! In a flash, I got up and went out the door, the cat, still hanging on the door when I opened it and closed it. I picked him off the door and carried him inside. My father still sitting stunned, said, "My God it's a cat. You can't keep that in here." Silently, I looked at him and smiled. I held Sam up to face my father and Sam stared at him directly pupils widening. Only Sam was unique. His left pupil expanded horizontally while his right one expanded vertically! It was then I also learned that spirit has a great sense of humor.

Sam stayed with me from then on. He'd sleep on my desk while I silently wrote poetry and had it published worldwide. Sam would go in the car with me on errands. And as if everyone who enjoyed a cat as a pet did this, Sam would go with me for long walks at the lake and sit on the sand mounds and look out at the lake with me. Sam was, in fact, the only one who seemed to understand me.

A Manifested Destiny

Eventually, I read every single book on metaphysics and spirituality that I could get my hands on. And within a few months, it'd be time for me to consider moving along to college. So, I took a job at a nursing home nearby. It was a kind of nursing home and hospice all in one. This position was perfectly suited to me. My compassion and love finally had a proper place to channel to, and the job was a fun training ground for the things I had just come to learn.

As I got to know the patients and their level of ailments, I also realized I could sense and feel their feelings, their needs, and their dead relatives that stood with them day and night. Soon I was able to detect and feel when people would be passing because the relatives would come nearer, and I would feel this. This ability to sense such events didn't sadden me or scare me but instead comforted me because I already 'knew' these events were coming. My job was to comfort and aid the patient in my limited duties though my words and connection with them were never limited. The patients, whom I remember clearly even today, connected with me and understood as they neared their end, that I understood and was holding a loving space for them as they transitioned into spirit. I found this to be a very loving experience and one that would later prepare me for my healing work as a medical intuitive, helping people connect with those who've passed on in order to heal their relationships, or gain comfort that they were indeed, settled and at peace.

For me, taking six months of silence was a blessing that we don't often get to do in life, and it allowed me to build and grow into the Mastery I have today for both healing and medical intuition. As an Indigo child, I was on the second tier of souls who came in to hold the light and show the way for others. If I had to do it all over again, I wouldn't change a thing. Everything, including Sam, was a blessing because I was willing to take time to learn, listen, and grow. From that, arose a new destiny manifested.

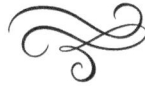

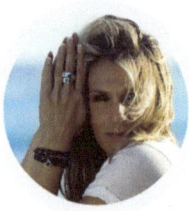

Winifred Adams, Professional Wellness Speaker, Radio Show Host, Medical Intuitive, Master Healer, Best-Selling Author, Award-Winning Musician, Jewelry Designer.

Winifred is a Medical Intuitive/Master Healer, Radio Show Host, and Professional Wellness Speaker for Making Life Brighter. Finding the origin of energetic imbalances, Winifred's rare, but vast skill set shifts energy in Live-Time™, creating an environment for complete healing. Winifred, shares her rare gifts of intuition with audiences, creating an experience of Live-Time Healing™. Hire Winifred to speak to your audience.

Connect with Winifred:

www.makinglifebrighter.com

This page is intentionally left blank

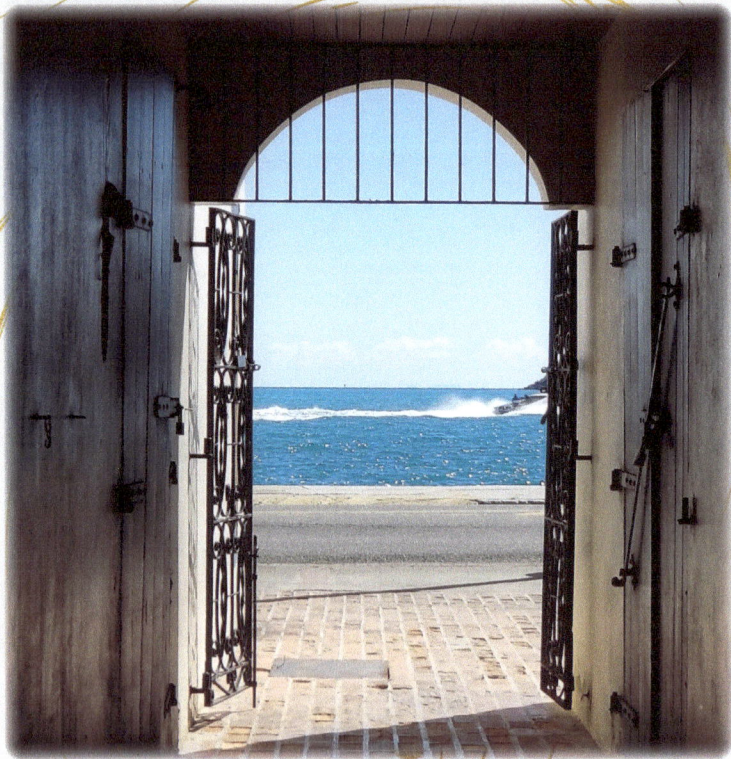

As We Leave You

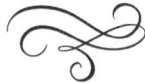

*I*T HAS BEEN such an honor to share these amazing stories with you, and it has especially been my incredible blessing to have the opportunity to introduce you to each of the authors whose stories you have had the cherished pleasure of reading within the covers of this little book.

There are journeys that we embark on sometimes which allows us to believe we are doing something to help others transform their lives. But it is just as often that those journeys also end up allowing us to transform as well. Such is the case with the journey I undertook with this little book which began in October 2018 in Costa Rica. Someday, perhaps I will tell you the story behind Manifested Blessings beginnings, but for now, I would like to leave you with just one of the lessons I learned while on this journey to bring this little book and it's wonderful author's stories to you.

Simply put, it's to be the change you wish to see around you. By demonstrating what it is that you desire to have in your life, through words, actions, even in-actions, and through each choice that you make. By demonstrating what it is you are willing to accept in your world, you are helping others to learn from your example. By watching as you gently walk upon this Earth, living and conducting your life in the way in which you desire others to be with you, you are lending your wisdom and your heart to the healing journey that our world and humanity is currently on.

By demonstrating through our own words, actions, and mannerisms how we choose to step through life, we are gently and lovingly allowing others to adopt our ways and in doing so, we are, one by one, creating change that allows us all to Manifest a life and a world we desire to see exist.

One of the most valuable lessons I've learned while bringing this book to you can be summed up in a single sentence shared by Dr. Paul Leon Masters. "For all I know I know nothing, if I cannot demonstrate a better life."

May the life you desire to manifest demonstrate to the world around you that you are indeed living your best life and doing so from the inside out for all to witness and emulate if they choose.

If you loved this book and have a story you would like to share in our next Volume of Manifested Blessings, or one of our upcoming Anthologies, using the QR-Code below, visit our site to learn more.

https://carnelianmoonpublishing.com/work-with-us/anthologies-collection

We look forward to bringing you more stories soon! Until then, we are waiting to welcome you to our sites!

https://carnelianmoonpublishing.com
https://carnelianmoonpublishing.com/anthologies-collection
https://theinspiredlivingacademy.newzenler.com

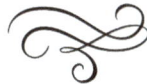

Book Development Credits

Deborah's Story: Heart love puzzle missing part by PIRO4D. https://pixabay.com/illustrations/heart-love-puzzle-missing-part-1745300/

Debbie: Mother Baby Love Sunset Beach by by Mohamed Hassan. https://pixabay.com/illustrations/mother-baby-love-sunset-beach-4475732/

Mary: Dog Cavalier King Charles Spaniel by Alexas_Fotos. https://pixabay.com/photos/dog-cavalier-king-charles-spaniel-762518/

Cathy: World globe worldwide children by Prawny. https://pixabay.com/illustrations/world-globe-worldwide-www-global-1302959/

Winifred: Hand butterfly clouds flying by by Geralt.   https://pixabay.com/photos/hand-butterfly-clouds-flying-3751159/

Cover photo by Judith Richardson Schroeder - St. Thomas Bahamas, 2018

Cover Design by Trevor Thomas, LightWerx Media

Interior Design & Layout by Simon Brimble

www.ingramcontent.com/pod-product-compliance
Lightning Source LLC
Chambersburg PA
CBHW041242020426
42333CB00003B/56